EXERCISES AND HABITS TO IMPROVE YOUR EYESIGHT

How to Improve Your Eyesight Naturally And Use Eye Exercises to Improve Vision

James Edwards

TABLE OF CONTENTS

INTRODUCTION

Our eyes suffer greatly from continuous screen time, environmental stressors, and sedentary habits in the busyness of our modern lives. Our eyesight frequently suffers casualties as we navigate a world where digital devices rule, leaving us to deal with weariness, strain, and a progressive loss of visual acuity. The pursuit of better vision extends beyond achieving a normal vision; it also involves encouraging a proactive and comprehensive approach to eye health.

The extensive manual 'EXERCISES AND HABITS TO IMPROVE YOUR EYESIGHT' is intended to empower you on your path to ideal eyesight. Within these pages, we explore the realm of practices and workouts that can dramatically improve the condition and functionality of your eyes. This book is a guide to creating a lifestyle that enhances and maintains the health of your eyes, not just a list of methods to improve your vision.

'EXERCISES AND HABITS TO IMPROVE YOUR EYESIGHT' provides a comprehensive examination of techniques that can improve your vision naturally, ranging from focused eye exercises to mindful habits. This book offers useful insights and doable solutions for anyone looking to reduce eye strain, slow down age-related vision changes, or simply maintain vibrant eye health.

Come along on an adventure that goes beyond conventional methods of eye care. Learn how your lifestyle choices and the clarity of your vision are mutually beneficial. You'll discover an abundance of knowledge, backed by academic study, as we delve into the implications of eye health, pointing you in the direction of a more comprehensible and hopeful future.

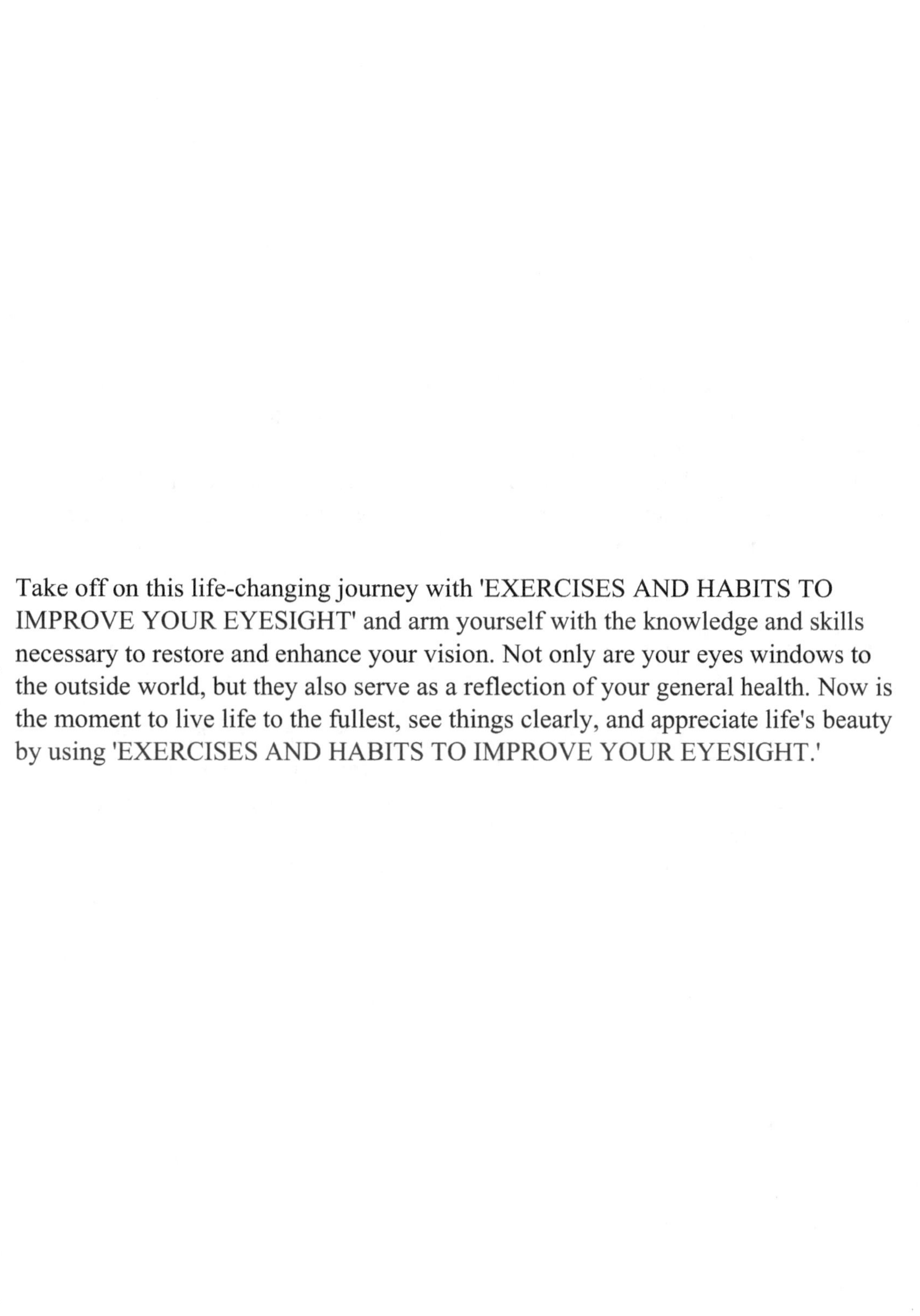

Take off on this life-changing journey with 'EXERCISES AND HABITS TO IMPROVE YOUR EYESIGHT' and arm yourself with the knowledge and skills necessary to restore and enhance your vision. Not only are your eyes windows to the outside world, but they also serve as a reflection of your general health. Now is the moment to live life to the fullest, see things clearly, and appreciate life's beauty by using 'EXERCISES AND HABITS TO IMPROVE YOUR EYESIGHT.'

<h1 style="text-align:center">CHAPTER ONE</h1>

<h1 style="text-align:center">The Connection Between Lifestyle and Eyesight</h1>

Our eyes are under unbelievable levels of strain in the fast-paced digital age where screens rule our daily lives and convenience frequently takes precedence over health. There has been an increase in vision-related problems as a result of the widespread use of digital devices, sedentary lifestyles, and poor eating habits. The good news is that maintaining and enhancing our vision is greatly influenced by the lifestyle decisions we make.

The Problem of Digital Age to Eyesight

The way we work, communicate and pass our time has changed due to the widespread use of computers, smartphones, and other digital devices. Unfortunately, our eyes suffer from a unique set of problems as a result of our continuous screen exposure. Extended periods of time spent in front of a computer can result in digital eye strain, which manifests as headaches, dry eyes, and blurred vision.

The Value of Breaks and Blinking for Healthy Eyes:

We frequently neglect to give our eyes the breaks they require in our pursuit of productivity. The 20-20-20 rule is a straightforward but powerful eye strain prevention method. Take a 20-second break and concentrate on something 20 feet away for every 20 minutes you spend staring at a screen. Consciously blinking also keeps the eyes from drying out by keeping them moist.

Eating Right for Optimal Vision

In addition to being good for general health, a nutrient-rich, well-balanced diet is essential for maintaining eye health. Foods rich in zinc and other minerals, along with vitamins A, C, and E, help to keep the eyes healthy. Rich in omega-3 fatty acids, colorful fruits, and leafy greens are especially good for you.

Hydration and the Health of Your Eyes:

It's common to forget about proper hydration when discussing eye health. Maintaining proper hydration lowers the chance of dry eyes by keeping the eyes sufficiently lubricated. Maintaining optimal eye function can be achieved with a simple yet effective habit of drinking water throughout the day.

Exercise and Blood Flow:

Frequent exercise has a positive impact on eye health in addition to being vital for general well-being. Healthy blood circulation is facilitated by exercise, and this is essential for providing the eyes with oxygen and nutrients. Furthermore, exercises like walking outside that require you to focus on objects at different distances can help strengthen and exercise your eye muscles.

The Function of Sleep

Good sleep is essential for overall health, and its effects on eye health are significant. The eyes have a chance to relax and heal while they sleep. Insufficient sleep can result in various negative conditions such as dry eyes and eye fatigue. Maintaining good vision depends on developing a regular sleep schedule and a comfortable sleeping environment.

Techniques for Eye Relaxation and Mindfulness:

One of the major experience we witness in the busy digital age era we live is stress. Tension and eye strain are just two ways that stress can appear. Deep breathing and eye exercises are examples of mindfulness and relaxation techniques that you can incorporate into your routine to help reduce stress and encourage a calm state for your eyes.

In summary, our vision is a priceless gift that needs to be carefully preserved and improved. Our eyesight can be greatly improved and preserved by leading mindful lifestyles that prioritize sleep, manage screen time, eat a nutrient-rich diet, stay hydrated, exercise frequently, and practice relaxation techniques. This chapter is a groundwork to help you take charge of your lifestyle and develop habits that will support the longevity of your visual health as well as your general well-being.

CHAPTER TWO

The Fundamentals of Eye Structure and Function

An understanding of the structure and function of the eyes is essential when trying to improve vision through exercise and habit. The eyes are complex organs that are essential to how we see the outside world. The fundamentals of eye anatomy will be covered in this chapter, along with an exploration of the various structures and their purposes.

The Outer Frameworks of the Eyes

1. Sclera and Cornea:

The transparent front portion of the eye that covers the anterior chamber, pupil, and iris is called the cornea. It helps focus light onto the retina and serves as a barrier of defense. The sclera, also referred to as the white of the eye, keeps the eyeball shaped and provides structural support.

2. The conjunctiva

The thin, transparent membrane that covers the sclera and inner eyelids is called the conjunctiva. It keeps foreign objects out of the eye and helps lubricate it.

3. Eyelids and Eyelashes:

The eyes are shielded from dust and bright light by the eyelids. In contrast, eyelashes serve as sensors that cause the eyelids to reflexively close in response to external stimuli.

4. Tear glands:

The tear glands secrete tears in order to lubricate the eyes and remove irritating substances. Retaining tear production requires adequate hydration.

The Inner Frameworks of the Eyes

1. Iris and Pupil:

The amount of light that enters the eye through the pupil is controlled by the iris, the colored portion of the eye. The size of the pupil changes in response to the focus of the eye and the lighting.

2. Lens

The lens aids in focusing light onto the retina and is situated behind the iris. Enhancing the flexibility of the eye muscles through exercise can help with accommodation and focus.

3. The retina

Photoreceptors, which include rods and cones, are specialized cells found in the retina that transform light into signals that are transmitted to the brain through the optic nerve. Frequent ocular exercises can improve these cells' efficiency.

4. Optic Nerve

The retina sends visual data to the brain through the optic nerve. A few routines can help the optic nerve function at its best for better signal transmission.

The Significance of Blood Flow

Having enough blood flow is essential to keeping the eyes healthy. A balanced diet, regular exercise, and adequate hydration all help to promote optimal blood flow, which supplies the eyes with the nutrients they need for maximum health and repair.

Exercise and Lifestyle Suggestions

1. Eye Motions:

Practice focusing on close and far objects, rolling your eyes in all directions, and tracing imaginary shapes with your eyes. These exercises improve muscle flexibility in the eyes.

2. Palming

After rubbing your hands together to create heat, lightly cup them over your closed eyes. This method of relaxation eases eye strain.

3. Exercises for Blinking:

Intentional blinking lessens dry eyes and lubricates the eyes. Make blinking exercises a daily habit, particularly if you spend a lot of time in front of screens.

4. Nutrition for Eye Comfort:

Eat a diet high in minerals like zinc and omega-3 fatty acids, as well as vitamins A, C, and E. These nutrients help maintain the health of the eyes and could lead to better vision.

Keep in mind that when using these exercises and habits, consistency is essential. Gaining knowledge of the intricate details of eye anatomy and function paves the way for improving your vision holistically by combining focused exercises with mindful habits.

CHAPTER THREE

Discover the Value of A Balanced Diet for Your Eyesight

Our eyes are complex, delicate organs that allow us to see the world around us. They are marvels of biological engineering. However, we sometimes overlook the basic role that nutrition plays in preserving the best possible eye health in the midst of the hustle and bustle of modern life. This chapter will examine the critical relationship that exists between the health of our eyes and a balanced diet, as well as the ways in which forming healthy eating habits can both protect and enhance your vision.

Important Vitamins and Minerals for Your Eyesight

Like every other part of our body, the eyes need a variety of nutrients in order to function at their best. The following are some of the vital vitamins and minerals needed for eye health:

1. Vitamin A: Because it is essential to the retina's proper functioning, this vitamin is essential for preserving good vision. Other vision issues, including night blindness, can result from a vitamin A deficiency.

2. Vitamin C: Well-known for strengthening the immune system, vitamin C also helps to keep the blood vessels in the eyes healthy and ward off diseases like cataracts.

3. Vitamin E: Being a potent antioxidant, vitamin E promotes general eye health by shielding the eyes from oxidative damage.

4. Zinc: A zinc deficiency has been related to impaired night vision. Zinc is necessary for the appropriate function of enzymes in the eye.

5. Omega-3 Fatty Acids: Rich in walnuts, flaxseeds, and fish, omega-3 fatty acids are essential for preserving the retina's structural integrity and advancing general eye health.

Color Your Plate with Different Nutrients

Eat a diet high in vibrant fruits and vegetables because they are a great source of the vitamins and antioxidants that are necessary for healthy eyes. Add a range of orange and yellow fruits, such as mangoes and oranges, berries, such as blueberries and strawberries, and leafy greens, such as spinach and kale.

A Diet Plan for Good Eyesight

This is a short guide to creating an eye-healthy diet:

1. Leafy Greens: Rich in vitamins A, C, and E are spinach, kale, collard greens, and Swiss chard.

2. Multicolored Fruits and Vegetables: A variety of nutrients essential for eye health can be found in carrots, sweet potatoes, bell peppers, oranges, and berries.

3. Omega-3 Rich Foods: Include walnuts, flaxseeds, chia seeds, and fatty fish like salmon and mackerel in your diet.

4. Nuts and Seeds: Zinc and vitamin E are found in almonds, sunflower seeds, and hazelnuts, which support the general health of your eyes.

5. Lean Proteins: Since zinc is necessary to keep the retina healthy, include foods like chicken, eggs, and lean meats in your diet.

Consciously selecting a diet rich in a variety of nutrient-dense foods benefits your overall health in addition to maintaining the health of your eyes. Recall that eating a balanced diet is a comprehensive strategy for raising your quality of life, not just for vision improvement. Thus, relish the variety of a wholesome dish and observe your vision flourish.

CHAPTER FOUR

The Effect of Hydration on Your Eyesight

Dry eye syndrome is one of the most prevalent conditions linked to dehydration that affects the eyes. The body produces fewer tears when it doesn't have enough water, which can cause dryness, irritation, and discomfort. Mucus, oils, water, and antibodies are the components of tears that lubricate the eyes. This delicate balance is upset when there is insufficient water in the body, making the eyes more prone to irritation and inflammation.

Drinking Plenty of Water to Avoid Eye Fatigue

With our screen-centric, modern lifestyles, eye fatigue has become a common issue. Long-term screen staring can cause symptoms like headaches, blurry vision, and difficulty focusing. By promoting tear production and preserving the lubrication of the eyes, adequate hydration helps to prevent eye fatigue. The eyes are better able to withstand extended amounts of screen time without strain when they are properly hydrated.

Advice on Staying Hydrated for Good Eye Health

1. Stay Hydrated: Make an effort to ensure that you consume a sufficient amount of water throughout the day. Keep a water bottle on you as a constant reminder to drink plenty of water.

2. Balanced Diet: Eat a lot of foods high in water, like fruits and vegetables. These foods supply vital vitamins and minerals that are good for eye health in addition to aiding with general hydration.

3. Limit Dehydrating Beverages: Cut back on the amount of liquids you consume, such as alcohol and caffeinated drinks, as these can cause dehydration. These drinks may cause you to lose more fluids and may harm your eyes.

4. Use Artificial Tears: To temporarily relieve and maintain moisture in situations where extended screen time or environmental factors may contribute to dry eyes, think about using artificial tears.

In summary, maintaining adequate hydration is essential for good health and should have a significant effect on vision. You can actively support the health of your eyes by making adequate hydration a priority through mindful water consumption, a balanced diet, and minimizing dehydrating factors. You will probably notice improvements in your general vitality and well-being as well as in the health of your eyes as you make drinking water a regular part of your routine.

CHAPTER FIVE

The Power of Sleep to Improve Your Eyesight

We frequently concentrate on exercises, habit changes, and lifestyle adjustments in our quest for better vision. Even though these are unquestionably important, getting enough sleep is an unsung hero in the quest for better vision. This chapter explores the significant effects that restorative sleep can have on preserving and even improving vision.

A well-rested mind guides the eyes, which are windows to the soul. The brain is intricately linked to our eyes, which are sophisticated and complex organs. Visual information is transmitted from the eyes to the brain via the optic nerve, where it is processed and interpreted. A rested mind guarantees that the complex neural networks that power vision operate at their best.

How Sleep Restores the Health of Our Eyes

The body goes through vital processes of renewal and repair during each stage of sleep. This translates to the eyes in terms of cell regeneration, tissue repair, and the generation of essential fluids that maintain the eyes' moisture and nourishment. This natural healing process is affected negatively by insufficient sleep, which can result in dry eyes, eye strain, and other vision-related problems.

Melatonin: The Sleep Hormone's Effect on the Health of Your Vision

Melatonin is essential for preserving eye health and is frequently linked to the regulation of sleep-wake cycles. This hormone, which is generated while you sleep, functions as a potent antioxidant that shields your eyes from oxidative damage. Not only does getting enough sleep allow your body to recuperate, but it also helps your body produce melatonin, which incidentally protects your vision.

Digital Eye Strain: A Current Illness That Needs a Restful Night's Sleep

Many people in this day and age of technology spend a lot of time staring at screens. Digital eye strain is a condition that has emerged in this digital age. In this context, getting enough sleep is even more important because it helps prevent and treat the symptoms of prolonged screen time, like dry eyes, blurred vision, and eye fatigue.

How to Create a Sleep Schedule for Better Eyesight

1. Consistent Bedtime: Adhere to a regular sleep schedule by going to bed at the same time every day. This improves the quality of your sleep by balancing your body's internal clock.

2. Establish a Calm Bedtime Routine: Before going to bed, conduct peaceful activities like reading a book, having a warm bath, or doing relaxation techniques. Your body will receive this as a cue to wind down.

3. Adjust Your Sleep Environment to Encourage Better Sleep: Make sure your bedroom is cool, quiet, and dark to promote restful sleep. Make an effort to get a comfortable pillow and mattress to assist you in enjoying better sleep at night.

In conclusion, don't undervalue the importance of getting a good night's sleep in the quest for better vision. You can give your eyes the best possible environment for healing, regeneration, and protection by prioritizing good sleep. Sleeping well has many rejuvenating benefits, so keep that in mind as you incorporate habits and exercises into your daily routine to improve your eyesight.

CHAPTER SIX

Popular Exercises to Improve Your Eyesight

Our eyes often suffer as a result of the fast-paced, screen-dominated lifestyle of the digital age. But just as we exercise our bodies to stay in shape, we also need to include eye-friendly exercises in our regimens to preserve and enhance our vision. The goals of these exercises are to increase flexibility, reduce eye strain, and improve overall visual acuity.

1. The Palming Method

A quick and efficient way to ease strained eyes and lower stress is to practice palming. Look for a peaceful spot to sit. After giving your hands a good rub to produce heat, cup your palms and gently place them over your closed eyes without pressing. Take a deep breath, and let your palms' warmth comfort your eyes. To increase the level of relaxation, picture a serene setting, like a lush forest or a calm beach. To rejuvenate your eyes, practice palming for five to ten minutes every day.

2. Shifting Attention

Flexibility and the ability to focus on both close and far objects are enhanced by this exercise. Pick a nearby object and give it your whole attention for a short while. After that, turn your attention to a far-off object and stare at it for a short while longer. Keep switching between close and far objects while progressively extending the distance. To improve your eye's focusing abilities, repeat this exercise for five to ten minutes.

3. The Eye Movement in Figure 8

This exercise increases flexibility and eye coordination. Imagine that ten feet or so in front of you is a big figure eight, representing infinity. With your eyes, trace the imaginary number eight, going slowly and fluidly. After two to three minutes, reverse your direction and follow the shape of the eight. Maintaining an ideal eye movement range and enhancing eye coordination are two benefits of this exercise.

4. Magnifying

Exercises that zoom in are good for keeping your eye muscles flexible. Hold an object at arm's length, it could be your thumb or something small. After a short while, keep your attention on the object and gradually bring it closer to your eyes. Keep moving the object back and forth while progressively quickening your pace. Take two to three minutes to complete this exercise to improve your eyes' ability to focus.

5. Blinking Exercises

Although blinking is frequently disregarded, it is essential for preserving eye moisture and lowering dryness. For two minutes, blink quickly as the timer counts down. This exercise helps you avoid the pain that comes with spending too much time in front of a screen.

6. The 20-20-20 Guideline

Our eyes are constantly exposed to screens in the digital age, which causes eye fatigue and strain. The 20-20-20 rule can help combat this. It states that you should look at something 20 feet away and take a 20-second break every 20 minutes. This little break helps you avoid digital eye strain by allowing your eyes to rest and focus again.

It's important for you to include these exercises that are good for your eyes in your daily routine to help with eye strain and improve your eyesight. To maintain the long-term health of your eyes, it is imperative that you become consistent with these exercises. Your general vision and well-being will probably improve as you build up your eye muscles and practice more mindful eye care.

CHAPTER SEVEN

Avoiding Digital Eye Strain in A Digital Age Era

In our technologically advanced, fast-paced world, we are spending more and more time in front of screens. Our eyes are continually subjected to the harsh glare of screens, whether we're using a computer, browsing social media on our phones, or binge-watching our favorite TV series. A condition known as Digital Eye Strain (DES), which can cause discomfort and possibly have long-term effects on your eyesight, can result from this prolonged exposure. This chapter will explain digital eye strain, discuss its symptoms, and — most importantly — show you how to avoid it by adopting a few easy-to-follow habits.

Recognizing Digital Eye Strain

One common ailment that results from using digital devices for extended periods of time is digital eye strain. There is a wide range of symptoms that can include:

1. Eye discomfort: itching, redness, or a scratchy feeling in the eyes.

2. Blurry Vision: Inability to focus on objects after prolonged use of a screen.

3. Headaches: Chronic headaches that frequently begin in the forehead and temple area.

4. Shoulder and Neck Pain: strained muscles from using digital devices with bad posture.

5. Sleep Disturbances: Screen exposure can disrupt sleep cycles by emitting blue light.

The 20-20-20 Guideline

The 20-20-20 rule is one practical strategy to avoid digital eye strain. Take a 20-second break and concentrate on something 20 feet away for every 20 minutes you spend staring at a screen. You can lessen eye strain and relax your eye muscles by adopting this easy habit.

Correct Lighting and Workplace Design

Establish a cozy, well-lit workstation. To ease shoulder and neck strain, adjust your computer screen to eye level. To lessen the glare on your screen, use ambient lighting. If necessary, you may also want to use an anti-glare filter.

Blink Often

Dry eyes can result from a decrease in blink rates brought on by prolonged screen staring. Try to blink frequently to avoid dry eyes and maintain moisture in your eyes.

Modify the Display Configuration

You can change the font size, contrast, and screen brightness on the majority of digital devices. Make the most of these settings to ensure a satisfying viewing experience. In addition, you might want to use your device's "night mode" feature, which lowers the emission of blue light at night.

Computer Eyewear

Make an investment in anti-reflective computer glasses. The purpose of these glasses is to lessen glare and eye strain when using screens for extended periods of time.

Frequent Ocular Examinations

See an optometrist for routine eye exams to keep an eye on the health of your eyes. Make sure your prescription is current if you currently wear glasses, as an out-of-date prescription can exacerbate eye strain.

Exercise to Maintain Eye Health

Include eye exercises in your everyday schedule. Easy exercises like concentrating on a close object first and then a far away one can ease eye strain and strengthen the eye muscles.

A Time of Digital Withdrawal

Think about including a digital detox in your daily routine. Set aside specified periods of time each day to completely unplug from screens. Take advantage of this time to read a book in print, go outside, or just unwind without being distracted by technology.

You can greatly lower your chance of developing digital eye strain and preserve good eye health by forming these habits and being aware of how much time you spend in front of the screen. In the digital age, taking preventative measures to safeguard your vision is crucial to your overall health.

CHAPTER EIGHT

Outdoor Activities to Improve Your Eyesight

Our eyes are continuously exposed to artificial lighting, digital screens, and indoor environments in our screen-dominated modern world. Our eyesight can suffer from this sedentary lifestyle, which can lead to eye strain, weariness, and even long-term vision issues. Nonetheless, there is a straightforward but effective way to mitigate these effects: spending more time outside participating in activities that improve our general health and sight.

1. Advantages of Sunlight for Eyesight:

There are numerous advantages that natural sunlight has for your eyes. The circadian rhythm, your body's internal clock, is regulated by exposure to sunlight. This, in turn, affects your sleep patterns and general well-being. In terms of vision, sunlight causes the retina's dopamine to release, which is a neurotransmitter necessary for keeping eyesight in a healthy state.

Aim to spend a minimum of 20 to 30 minutes outside every day, allowing yourself to absorb the natural sunlight.

Take brief breaks from your computer work to go outside and let the natural light soothe your eyes.

2. Distance Vision Practice:

Computer vision syndrome is a condition that can result from prolonged screen staring. Engage in activities that improve your distance vision to offset this. Your eyes can strengthen and adjust to a variety of focal points and depths found in outdoor environments.

Go outside and do things like hiking, bird watching, or just taking a leisurely stroll in a park that requires you to focus on far-off objects.

3. The Rule of 20-20-20:

In order to reduce eye strain and stop the progression of myopia, adhere to the 20-20-20 rule. Every 20 minutes, take a 20-second break and focus your gaze 20 feet away. This rule works best in outdoor environments because the natural landscape offers a variety of visual stimuli.

When engaging in outdoor activities, set a timer to serve as a constant reminder to adhere to the 20-20-20 rule.

4. Visually Pleasing Sports:

Playing sports enhances eye health in addition to general fitness. Playing sports requiring quick eye movements, such as badminton, tennis, or even a casual game of catch, improves hand-eye coordination.

Make sure your routine includes sports where you have to keep track of moving objects quickly. This can entail engaging in sports like soccer, tennis, or even frisbee throwing.

5. Relaxation and Mindful Breathing:

Tension and stress can show up in your eyes, impairing your vision. Engaging in outdoor activities offers a fantastic environment for practicing mindfulness and relaxation techniques, like deep breathing and meditation.

Locate a peaceful outdoor area to practice meditation and deep breathing, ideally in the middle of nature. This may lessen strained eyes and encourage general relaxation.

Taking part in these outdoor activities improves your physical health and helps maintain the health of your eyes. Make a deliberate effort to balance outdoor activities with screen time, and your eyes will appreciate the welcome shift. Recall that maintaining good eye health is a lifestyle decision that will benefit your eyesight by allowing you to see more clearly and healthily.

CHAPTER NINE

Supplements and Nutrients for Improving Your Eyesight

We frequently concentrate on routines and exercises in our quest for better vision, but it's just as crucial to nourish our eyes internally. Proper nutrition and supplementation are essential for both preserving and improving vision. Important components that can lead to better vision and overall eye health are examined in this chapter.

Important Nutrients for Eye Health

1. Vitamin A

To keep your eyes healthy and avoid night blindness, you need to take vitamin A. Kale, sweet potatoes, spinach, and carrots are among the foods high in vitamin A. By incorporating these into your diet, you can enhance your vision in low light and maintain the health of your retina.

2. Omega-3 Fatty Acids

Omega-3 fatty acids, which are abundant in fatty fish like salmon, trout, and sardines, support the structural integrity of the eye. These lipids are essential for preserving the health of the retinas and avoiding dry eyes. Consider taking fish oil capsules or other omega-3 supplements if you're not a big fish fan.

3. Zeaxanthin and Lutein

Lutein and zeaxanthin are antioxidants that shield the eyes from damaging high-energy light waves like ultraviolet rays. The retina contains large amounts of them. Corn, egg yolks, and leafy greens are excellent providers of these nutrients.

4. Vitamins E and C

These antioxidants help shield against vision issues brought on by aging. Vitamin C is abundant in citrus fruits, strawberries, almonds, and sunflower seeds; meanwhile, nuts, and seeds, are excellent providers of vitamin E, as are vegetable oils.

Supplements to Promote Eye Health

1. Extract from Bilberries

Strong antioxidants called anthocyanosides, found in bilberries, may lessen eye fatigue and enhance night vision. If you would like to supplement your diet, think about bilberries.

2. Zinc

High concentrations of zinc are found in the eye, especially in the retina. It aids in the conversion of beta-carotene into vitamin A, which is essential for eye health. Add foods high in zinc, such as beef, oysters, and pumpkin seeds, to your diet, or think about taking supplements.

3. Calcium

A possible connection between vitamin D deficiency and visual issues has been suggested by recent research. Spend time in the sun, eat foods high in vitamin D, such as fatty fish and fortified dairy products, and, if necessary, think about taking supplements.

Crafting a Diet Plan That Is Good for Your Eyesight

Creating a diet plan that is well-rounded and incorporates a range of fruits, vegetables, lean proteins, and whole grains will guarantee that you get all the nutrients your eyes need. Speak with a nutritionist or other medical expert to create a plan that works for your unique requirements and way of life.

Hydration Is Important for Eye Health

Maintaining proper hydration is essential for good general health, which includes eye health. Maintaining proper hydration guarantees that your eyes get the moisture they need to perform at their best. To keep your eyes healthy, stay hydrated throughout the day by drinking lots of water.

In summary, a healthy lifestyle that includes the appropriate nutrients and supplements can greatly enhance vision. To maintain and improve your eyesight, incorporate these dietary choices with the activities and routines covered in previous chapters. Recall that the best outcomes in eye care come from a comprehensive approach.

CHAPTER TEN

Effect of Stress on Your Eyesight

Stress has become an inevitable part of our daily lives in the fast-paced, modern world that we live in. Stress has a substantial impact on the eyes because they are among the most delicate and important organs. This chapter will examine the complex relationship between stress and eyesight and explain how managing your stress effectively can help you see better.

The Link Between the Eye and Brain

The eyes and brain are not separate entities; rather, they are intimately connected. Stress hormones like cortisol are released by the body as a natural reaction to stress, and these hormones can affect many body functions, including eyesight. Extended periods of stress can cause eye strain, blurred vision, and even aggravate pre-existing conditions like astigmatism or myopia (nearsightedness).

Recognizing Eye Strain

Prolonged screen time, a sedentary lifestyle, and stress are common causes of eye strain. Extended periods of time spent staring at screens or performing close-up tasks can cause eye muscle fatigue, which can cause headaches, discomfort, and blurred vision. In order to stop the cycle of eye strain and advance general eye health, stress management is crucial.

Techniques for Eye Relaxation

1. Palming: To create a warm, dark environment, close your eyes and cover them with your palms. This easy method can be especially helpful when taking breaks from work or studying to help relax the muscles in the eyes.

2. Eye Exercises: To strengthen your eyes and sharpen your focus, include eye exercises in your daily routine. Basic techniques such as eye rotations, focusing on both nearby and faraway objects, and practicing blinking can have a big impact.

3. Mindfulness Meditation: An overburdened mind is frequently the source of stress. In addition to lowering stress, mindfulness meditation encourages relaxation in every part of the body, including the eyes. Frequent practice will improve your concentration and reduce eye strain.

Exercise and Eye Health

Exercise significantly improves general well-being and reduces stress. Frequent exercise increases blood flow, lowers inflammation, and encourages the body's natural mood enhancers, endorphins, to be released. Better oxygen and nutrition reach the eyes as a result, supporting their optimal operation.

Habits for Maintaining Good Eyesight

1. The 20-20-20 Rule: Adhere to this guideline to avoid eye strain when using screens for extended periods of time. Every 20 minutes, take a 20-second break and focus your gaze 20 feet away. This little break aids with focus maintenance and eye muscle relaxation.

2. Appropriate Lighting: Make sure your work area is well-lit, and keep reflections and glare off of your screen. An easier time seeing and less eye strain are two benefits of proper lighting.

3. Balanced Nutrition: The general health of your eyes is influenced by a diet high in vitamins and minerals, especially those that are good for your eyes (zinc, vitamins A, C, and E). Add fish, colorful fruits, and leafy greens to your diet.

In summary, better vision involves more than just visual exercises. You can provide a comprehensive approach to preserving and improving your eyesight by implementing stress management techniques into your daily routine. A clear, vibrant vision that can withstand the demands of the modern world is built on a foundation of mental and physical well-being as well as healthy habits. Recall that maintaining good eye health is an investment in your general health and well-being that should be made for the rest of your life.

CHAPTER ELEVEN

Building Habits into Your Daily Life to Improve Your Eyesight

One of the most important things we can do to succeed in our quest for better eyesight through exercise and habit is to incorporate these activities into our everyday lives. Habits are effective instruments that, when used wisely, can result in long-lasting improvements. We will look at practical ways to incorporate eye exercises and good habits into your daily routine in this chapter.

1. Establish a Routine: It's important to commit your eye exercises to a daily schedule. Select times during the day when you can commit to doing these exercises for a few uninterrupted minutes. Regularity is essential, whether it's in the morning, at lunch, or right before bed.

2. Start Small and Increase Gradually: Start your eye exercises for a reasonable amount of time. It's critical to refrain from overcommitting yourself at first. Increase the duration and intensity of the exercises gradually as you get used to the program. This methodical approach guarantees sustained adherence and helps avert burnout.

3. Integrate Habits: To generate synergies, combine your eye exercises with current routines. For example, include eye exercises in this routine if you already practice mindfulness or meditation. Making connections between eye exercises and well-established routines facilitates their retention and integration into everyday routines.

4. Make Use of Triggers: Determine what sets you off to perform your eye exercises. A particular occasion, like taking a computer break, or a visual cue, like a sticky note on your desk, could serve as the trigger. Triggers serve as a strong link between the habit and its environment by serving as reminders.

5. Set Achievable Objectives: Establish attainable objectives for your eye exercise program. Unrealistic expectations can cause dissatisfaction and low motivation. As you go, acknowledge your little accomplishments and work your way up to more difficult objectives. The possibility of forming a habit is increased by this positive reinforcement.

6. Incorporate Social Support: Tell your friends, family, and coworkers about your resolve to improve your eyesight. Support networks can offer accountability and motivation. In order to promote a feeling of community and common objectives, think about taking part in group challenges or activities pertaining to eye health.

7. Adjust to Your Lifestyle: Make sure your eye exercises are well-suited to your daily routine. Include eye exercises that you can perform at your desk if your job requires a lot of sitting down. If you lead an active lifestyle, think about engaging in outdoor activities like hiking or nature walks that can help maintain good eye health.

8. Monitor Your Progress: To keep track of your progress, use a specific app or keep a journal. Keeping track of your accomplishments and noting any visual gains can be very motivating. Frequent introspection about your experience serves to reaffirm the beneficial effects of your routines.

9. Remain Adaptable: Since life is unpredictable, unanticipated events can throw off your schedule. Consider these disruptions as opportunities to learn and adapt rather than as setbacks. Gain the fortitude to modify your routines without completely giving them up.

10. Appreciate Consistency: The foundation of habit formation is consistency. Honor the days when you follow your schedule, even if it's only for a short while. These persistent efforts will eventually result in a noticeable improvement in your eyesight.

Through these habits, you can incorporate eye exercises into your daily routine to improve your eyesight and promote a well-rounded approach to overall health. Recall that improving your eyesight is a marathon, not a sprint, and the habits you form now will help you in the future.

CONCLUSION

We have now explored the strong link between healthy habits, exercise, and better eyesight. It is clear that taking a proactive approach to eye health can result in some amazing advantages. We have explored the complex relationship that exists between exercise, mindful practices, and improving our eyesight through the pages of this book.

As we've learned, the eyes are essential to our overall health rather than being separate, standalone objects. Regular exercise that targets the eye muscles and improves cardiovascular health, in general, can make a big difference in vision clarity. Long-term maintenance and improvement of eyesight also greatly depend on the development of sustainable habits, such as reducing screen time consciously, taking regular breaks for eye exercises, and eating a healthy diet.

Our experience has highlighted the value of perseverance and commitment in developing ocular health-promoting behaviors. We empower ourselves to lessen the negative effects of contemporary challenges on our vision by adopting habits that prioritize our eyes and integrating easy-to-do but effective exercises into our daily routines.

This book is a guide and a reminder that preventive steps can be taken to protect and improve our eyesight in a world where digital screens and sedentary lifestyles are commonplace. It is a call to action to take responsibility for our own visual health rather than just a prescription for exercise.

Let's start down the road toward a visual experience that is healthier and more vibrant now. May we experience the transformation of our eyesight as we incorporate physical activity and meaningful routines into our lives, and may we also enjoy the wider advantages that permeate every aspect of our lives. In the future, having clear vision will be more than just an optical feat; it will be a symbol of the coexistence of mindful living and our eyes' amazing resiliency.